GET FIT AND HEALTHY IN YOUR OWN HOME IN 20 MINUTES OR LESS

An Essential Daily Exercise Plan and Simple Meal Ideas to Lose Weight and Get the Body You Want

By Silvana Siskov

Thank you for purchasing
Get Fit and Healthy in Your Own Home in 20
Minutes or Less:
An Essential Daily Exercise Plan and Simple Meal
Ideas to Lose Weight and Get the Body You Want

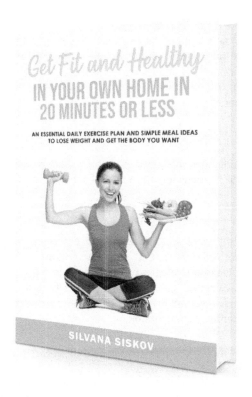

Go to bit.ly/silvana-recipebook to download
"Get Slim and Healthy in 20 Minutes or Less
Recipe Book,"
packed with delicious, simple and easy recipes,
to help you with your health and weight loss goals.

GET FIT AND HEALTHY IN YOUR OWN HOME IN 20 MINUTES OR LESS:
AN ESSENTIAL DAILY EXERCISE PLAN AND SIMPLE MEAL IDEAS TO LOSE
WEIGHT AND GET THE BODY YOU WANT
www.silvanasiskov.com

Table of Contents

Introduction

Two of the most common resolutions people make are to eat more healthily and to exercise more, usually in an effort to lose weight. These are also the two resolutions that people break most often, simply because they find them too hard to maintain.

They do not have to be that hard, however, keeping fit and maintaining a healthy diet are often seen by the vast majority of people as a sacrifice, instead of part of their self-care plan. Therefore, the resolution to eat and exercise regularly is easily broken.

If you have ever been in this situation, perhaps you have not approached it in the best way. For example, you may have assumed that keeping fit involves at least an hour at the gym or a five-mile run every day. While you can certainly do either of these, your exercise routine does not have to be like this.

If you are trying to fit an exercise regime into a busy lifestyle, you can do it in the comfort of your own home. Just 20 minutes a day will make a massive difference to your fitness levels, and you can even split that into two sessions of ten minutes each.

Similarly, healthy eating does not have to mean spending hours in the kitchen, preparing hard to obtain ingredients. You can easily make a wide range of healthy meals from a simple ingredients list, in as little as 20 minutes or less. This book will show you how to do this.

Eating well does not mean a limited range of bland recipes. The options are vast, and after you have been eating healthily for a while, you will wonder what you ever saw in fast food. Fad diets suck the energy out of you because your body is lacking essential nutrients. Eating healthy is different. It is the foundation for a good life. It is the choice that you make and it is something that you have full control of.

In the first two chapters of this book, you will learn the importance of both exercise and diet; the benefits of exercising and eating a healthy diet. You will be introduced to a variety of physical activities and healthy foods that can keep you in good health and support you on your journey to a healthy weight. You will also be shown how you can meet your goals in just 20 minutes or less.

In the next chapter, I will explain in more detail the kind of exercises you can do in the comfort of your own home. You will learn about warm-up exercises, how to exercise both your upper and lower body and how to get the most out of your stretching exercises.

Following that, you will receive some specific advice and plenty of simple ideas on how to prepare meals that are quick, healthy and delicious. Besides breakfast, lunch and dinner, we are going to look at how you can snack healthily throughout the day, as well as the best drinks to keep you fit and hydrated.

Finally, I will be giving you some advice on how to establish a routine that will allow you to stick to your healthy new lifestyle without it being a chore.

Getting fit and healthy does not have to be hard. You can do it in your own home in just 20 minutes or less; as long as you take the right approach.

In addition to all the great tips and meal ideas in this book, I am also offering you a free recipe book *Get Fit and Healthy in 20 Minutes or Less*. Go to bit.ly/silvana-recipebook and download your copy for free. You will receive a 29-page book, packed with healthy, simple and quick to prepare recipes. These recipes are designed to help you establish healthy habits, restore your energy levels and support your weight loss. The recipes are delicious and easy to prepare. The preparation time for each meal is only 20 minutes or less.

You will learn that healthy eating does not need to be difficult, expensive, time-consuming or tasteless. You will discover that with a little effort, you can achieve a healthy and fit body that you will feel proud of.

Chapter 1: Exercise

"Those who think they have no time for bodily exercise will sooner or later have to find time for illness."

Edward Stanley

Benefits of Exercising

Throughout most of human history, there was no need to build exercise into the daily routine, since people tended to live active lifestyles. Today, however, most of us travel by car, use labour-saving devices and sit down for most of our work and leisure activities.

That means that, whether we hit the gym or simply leave the car behind sometimes, it is vital to exercise consciously in a way that was unnecessary for our ancestors.

Exercising for Physical Health

According to the advice of the National Health Service (NHS) in the UK, "Whatever your age, there is strong scientific evidence that being physically active can help you lead a healthier and happier life." 150 minutes a week of moderate to vigorous-intensity activity has been shown to reduce the risk of many diseases. At the same time, extra exercise, such as playing sports or using the gym, intensifies this effect.

Exercises such as brisk walking, jogging, or cycling, for example, can reduce blood pressure and blood fat levels, as well as improve insulin sensitivity, body composition and cardiovascular fitness. These effects reduce the likelihood of developing the following conditions:

- Coronary heart disease and strokes (by 35%)
- Type 2 diabetes (by 50%)
- Various types of cancer (by 50%)
- Osteoarthritis (by 83%)
- Early death (by 30%)

This shows that including regular exercise into your life is a matter of priority and it is something that you must not ignore. Your health and the quality of your life greatly depend on it.

Exercising for Mental Health

Studies show that regular exercise can improve the brain's ability to handle stress and anxiety, as well as increasing the production of endorphins, which make you feel more positive. The overall effect is reduced stress and this seems to work even with a minimal amount of activity.

Regular exercise can also promote the growth of brain cells, especially in the hippocampus, the part of the brain that regulates memory and learning. It can not only improve general mental function as you grow older but may also reduce your risk of developing Alzheimer's disease.

Exercising for a Healthier Lifestyle

Besides fighting disease and promoting mental health, exercise can have a significant impact on your lifestyle. Of course, being healthier and feeling more positive can help you enjoy life more.

I love spending weekends going hiking. I do it whenever I can. It is such a pleasurable experience spending a day outdoors, enjoying the fresh air and being surrounded by the beauty of nature. I have adopted this activity as part of my life now and I love it.

I would like to encourage you to find an exercise you enjoy and then implement it into your routine. When it becomes routine, then it is something you do regularly. It becomes your lifestyle. You do not ask questions; you simply do it.

Exercise can also help you reduce weight, especially when you combine it with a healthy diet. It has also been proven to help with improving sleep, which underpins almost all aspects of a healthy lifestyle. We are all able to see the benefits of exercise for better sleep in children, as those who have been running around all day crash out and have a good night's sleep. In contrast, those who spend all day sitting and playing with their electronic devices often experience problems sleeping. The effect is similar, regardless of age.

Regular exercise can help you feel more energised, improve your mood and even boost your sex drive, allowing you to enjoy a fuller and more satisfying sex life. You can receive all these benefits from an activity that is not only easy to do but which you also enjoy.

What Is the Best Type of Exercise?

So, we have established that exercising has numerous benefits, but what kind of exercise should you be doing? Assuming you are aiming to maintain a healthy body and perhaps support your weight-loss diet, rather than hitting peak fitness for the Olympics or winning a body-building prize, there are various approaches.

A wide range of exercises can meet your needs, as long as you use them regularly. Ultimately, the best type of exercise is the one that you enjoy and feel comfortable doing. You will not notice the benefits of exercising if you do not like doing it or if you only do it once in a while. It is something that you need to implement regularly, so eventually exercise can become part of your routine. We will talk more about this in the last chapter of this book, which focuses on how to establish a healthy daily routine.

Now, let us look at the different types of physical activities that you can engage with.

Moderate Aerobic Activity

If you prefer not to push yourself too hard, approximately 150 minutes a week (that is about 20 minutes a day) of moderate aerobic activity, will usually be enough to keep you healthy and provide you with the benefits I mentioned before. This type of exercise should leave you slightly breathless, but you should still be able to speak effortlessly.

Moderate activity includes exercises such as brisk walking, cycling or dancing. And if you want your exercise to be useful in other ways, mowing the lawn or cleaning the house would count too. Swimming is also a valuable activity, especially if you are suffering from any type of joint pain, as the water buoys you up while you are active.

Vigorous-Intensity Activity

If you prefer to pack your activity into a shorter time, you will only need 75 minutes a week of vigorous-intensity activity for the same effect as 150 minutes at a moderate level. This type of physical activity will make you very breathless and prevent you from having a conversation. That is approximately ten minutes a day. Can you commit ten minutes of your time every day for the sake of having good health?

This type of activity can include running, speed cycling or hill cycling, as well as walking up a staircase. Sports that involve running, such as football, rugby or hockey, will count, as will gymnastics, martial arts or aerobics.

High-Intensity Interval Training (HIIT)

HIIT is an extra vigorous activity, alternating short bursts of intense anaerobic exercise with periods of moderate activity, such as walking (e.g. 30 seconds of intense exercise and 15 seconds of moderate exercise). It is important not to overdo HIIT. Sessions should certainly not be longer than 30 minutes at a time unless you are already extremely fit.

HIIT activities can include lifting heavy weights or circuit training. It can also involve interval running or sprinting up hills or stairs.

Muscle Strengthening Exercise

Muscle strengthening is not only for bodybuilders. It is a good idea to include it in any exercise regime. You can lift heavy weights, work with resistance bands or do press-ups or sit-ups, for instance, either in the gym or at home.

There are other ways of strengthening your muscles, such as doing yoga, tai-chi or pilates. Alternatively, you can simply take advantage of everyday opportunities, including digging your garden, carrying heavy shopping or even carrying tired kids. It all counts.

Doing any of these types of exercise on a regular basis can help you improve your health and maintain your fitness level.

Combining exercise with a healthy diet is the best way to achieve a healthy and fit body.

How to Get Fit in 20 Minutes or Less?

Daily exercise of 20 minutes does not sound like a lot, does it? In essence, it is not, and those 20 minutes can change your life.

Just 20 minutes of your day dedicated to exercise could lead to a healthier you. What this means is: weight loss, increased energy levels, a toned and lean body, a better mood, improved heart health and all manner of other benefits, which I am sure will be welcome in your life.

You can have all of these benefits in just 20 minutes.

How Do You Do It?

It is about having the right blend of exercise for you.

In this book, I have shared 25 exercises. They work with every part of your body, from your shoulders to your toes. You do not need to complete all of them every day. You can choose which exercises you want to do each day and you can select the most suitable time of the day to do them. I am sure just 20 minutes a day will be manageable to fit into your life, no matter how busy you are.

I want to warn you that if you have a particular injury or mobility problem, you should seek advice from your doctor or physio and tweak specific moves, so they do not harm or hurt you. All exercises can be modified. So, that is great news if you want to dedicate yourself to exercise and become fitter. Some exercises will require you to lift your leg high. If you feel pain in any part of your body, you might choose to lift your leg only halfway until your condition improves and you are able to challenge your body.

Try to start your workout with a few minutes of warm-up. It is important not to miss this step. Otherwise, you might end up with a muscle strain causing you some pain. Your warm-up can include running or jogging on the spot or jumping up and down. If you are unable to do any of these, then marching on the spot is a good alternative. You need to get your heart rate up and a little sweat going. Once you are feeling warm and your breathing is just a little faster than usual, you are ready to start working on each part of your body gradually.

It Is All About Toning

In the following chapter, we are going to cover some upper and lower body exercises that will not only work out the major muscles groups in each area but will keep the cardio element going. These exercises will also increase your flexibility and balance while at the same time working out your core.

The next chapter is about strength training. If you have some hand weights or small dumbbells, these will come in very handy and help you to tone your body a little faster. If you do not have these, a can of food will do the job just as well!

Once you finish your workout, spend the last few minutes cooling down with some stretches. You need to cool down your body just as much as you need to warm it up.

That is all it takes. Only 20 minutes of your day and over time you will start seriously noticing the difference. You will feel better, look fitter, and you will be healthier and stronger for it.

The good news is you do not need an expensive gym membership for this either, all you need is a little bit of floor space in the comfort of your own home!

Chapter 2: Get Fit In the Comfort of Your Home

"People find it hard to fit exercise into their working-day life. Nine to five jobs take up most of your day, so it is always difficult. But a little can go a long way. It can be 10 or 15 minutes of exercise that can be of real benefit."

Laura Trott

In this chapter, I will share with you five types of exercise that you can do in your own home. You will not need any type of gym equipment to do them properly and they can be easily performed by beginners and more advanced athletes. Some exercises will require you to use a chair or a bench or two cans of food instead of a set of dumbbells. You will not need to spend any money and you will not even need to leave your home. All you will need is the commitment to improve yourself.

There are 25 exercises organised into five groups, with five different exercises in each group. These five groups include warm-up exercises, upper body exercises, lower body exercises, strength training and stretching. All of them play important roles and work with different parts of your body.

This plan is flexible, and it does not require you to spend any money, it is not time-consuming, and it shows you how to get great results with exercising in less than 20 minutes a day.

There are some simple rules to follow:

- Do not stick to doing only one type of exercise every day. Each activity provides you with different kinds of benefits. So, make sure that over time, you include them all in your workout. Doing this can also help you reduce boredom and the risk of injury.
- You can choose to do two or three exercises from each exercise group one day and then different exercises the following day.
- You may decide to focus only on stretching exercises one or two days a week, to give your body a rest.
- Feel free to approach your new exercise regime whichever way suits you. You can choose to do your 20 minutes of exercising in the morning, or during your lunch break, or in the evening after work. You may decide to split this time into two parts and exercise for ten minutes in the morning and another ten minutes in the evening. The most important thing is to stay consistent. Do it regularly and do not give up.

The purpose of exercise is to make you feel good, and that is what you will achieve after you consistently repeat what I am teaching you. You will feel better, mentally and physically. You will also start to feel better about yourself. You will experience this only if you include exercise in your daily routine. Very soon you will notice the difference in the way you look and, most importantly, in the way you feel. Spending 20 minutes a day on self-care is not too long. It is only a small fraction of a day. Think about all the benefits that you can achieve within such a short period of time. I am sure that some days you may not feel like exercising, but I encourage you to do it anyway. Your body will thank you for it.

Warm-Up Exercises

Warm-up exercises prepare the body for exercise. They help increase the blood flow to your muscles and loosen your joints. They can prevent injuries, boost your metabolism and increase muscle temperature. They also increase your energy productions. Warm-up exercises are great for reducing muscle pain.

Running/Marching on the Spot

Warming up is vital, and one of the easiest ways to do this is to try running on the spot or marching. Anyone can do this. You can vary the intensity according to your general health and any injuries you may have that you are trying to protect.

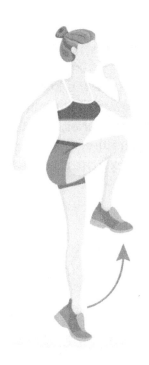

Benefits:

- Easy to do for anyone

- Warms up the body for cardiovascular exercise and strength training

- Works out all the major muscle groups

How to do it:

- Stand on the spot with your body upright and your shoulders back

- Start jogging or marching on the spot

- Lift your knees up as high as your hips

- Start to pump your arms up and down, moving them in the same rhythm as your feet

- Continue for 3 minutes

Knee Bends

You must protect your knees during any exercise. You can do this by bending your knees slightly whenever you do a workout on your lower body. However, warming up the muscles surrounding your knees is vital.

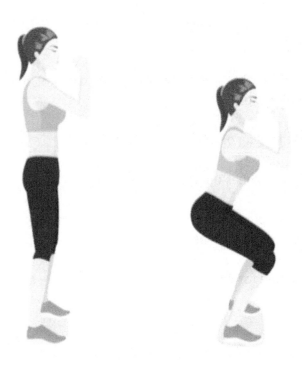

Benefits:

- Helps to warm up the muscles surrounding the knees

- Warms up the body for lower body exercise

- Raising your arms also warms up the upper body

- Easy to do

How to do it:

- Stand up straight with your legs shoulder-width apart and elbows bent

- Gently bend your knees, pushing your buttocks slightly back

- Do not bend your knees too much (see the picture)

- Slowly return to your standing position

- Repeat two sets 8-10 times

Jumping Jack

Jumping jack is a popular aerobic exercise and great for a total-body workout. It is an excellent fat burning exercise. I suggest you try to incorporate it into your morning routine. Doing so will help you get in shape and soon you will notice the difference to your fitness level.

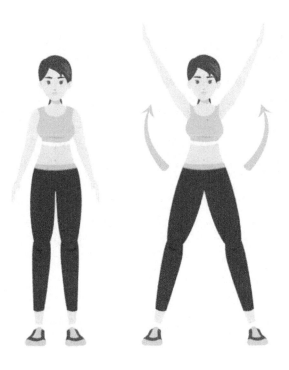

Benefits:

- Raises your heart rate and helps with weight loss

- Improves your mobility and circulation

- Works your heart, lungs and muscles

- Firms your glutes and calves

- Maintains your fitness level and helps you get in shape

- Helps you work on your biceps and triceps when slightly bending your arms

How to do it:

- Stand up straight with your legs together and arms at your sides

- Gently bend your knees and jump

- As you jump, spread your legs and stretch your arms as you can see in the picture

- Repeat this process for two minutes, try to do as many jumping jack's as you can during this time

- You can also repeat this jumping jack exercise several times a day for two minutes each time

Mountain Climber

This total-body workout is a great exercise for engaging your joints and muscles. It focuses on all of the body, from your neck down. Therefore, it works on many muscles at the same time. For this reason, it is a great warm-up exercise that can help you with your fitness level and overall health.

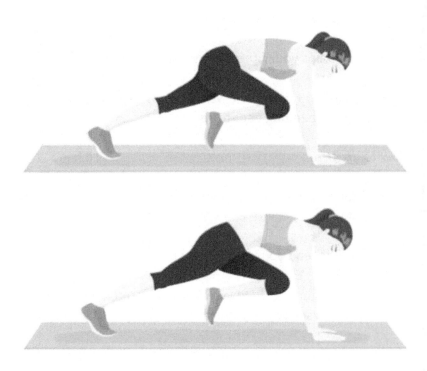

Benefits:

- Helps speed up your heart rate and supports the burning of calories and fat

- Helps with weight loss

- Helps build cardio endurance and strengthens the core

- Targets the abdominal muscles and builds triceps and shoulder muscles

- Works on quads and helps tone the glutes and hamstrings

How to do it:

- Lay down on your stomach, lift your body off the ground and keep your hips down

- Bring one knee to your chest, then pull it out

- Switch legs, and bring your other knee to your chest as much as you can, while you pull the other leg out

- Start slowly and then increase the speed, until you run against the floor

- Do a set of 10-15 in a row if you are a beginner and 25-30 if you are more advanced

Cross Body Toe Touches

This is an excellent exercise for people of any age and any fitness level. It involves many muscles, but it mainly focuses on the oblique muscle.

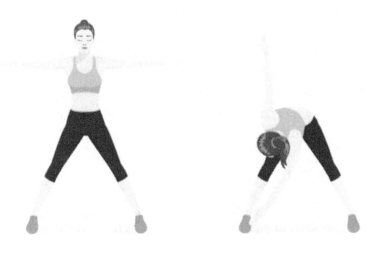

Benefits:

- Involves many muscles at the same time

- Works many muscles: obliques, shoulders, lower back, glutes and hamstring

- Great for your abdominal muscles and improving the strength of your core

- Stretches your back and hamstring

How to do it:

- Stand up straight with your legs shoulder-width apart

- Raise your arms to the sides as shown in the picture

- Bend down and touch your left toe with your right hand

- Keep rotating your body to the left and then to the right, reaching your toe with the opposite hand

- If you are not able to touch your toes, you can bend your knees slightly. The goal of this exercise is to rotate your body as fast as you can and squeeze your oblique muscle as hard as you can

- Do this exercise as fast as you can for one to two minutes

Upper Body Exercises

There are many health benefits of having a strong upper body. It can help heart health and improve your posture. A strong upper body plays a significant role in improving your flexibility and mobility as well as helping you to do a range of movements.

Shoulder Exercise – Power Partials

For this high-intensity exercise, you may want to get a set of dumbbells. These are easily available. If you do not have dumbbells, do not worry, you can use tins of food, which I am sure you can find in your kitchen cupboard. You simply need a small set of hand weights to work out your upper body and arms with ease.

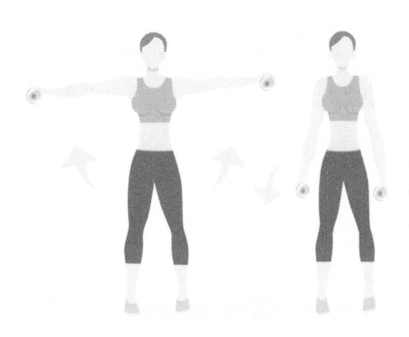

Benefits:

- Gives you a cardiovascular workout and helps with balance

- Engages the core muscles to add strength

- Focuses on the pectorals, the triceps and biceps

How to do it:

- Stand up straight with your feet shoulder-width apart and take your dumbbells/tins of food in your hands

- When you are ready, raise your arms out to the sides, level with your shoulders

- Hold the position for a few seconds and then lower your arms to your hips

- Repeat this process 12-15 times

- When you are ready to take this exercise to the next level and make it harder, instead of bringing your arms down to your hips, raise your arms straight above your head, hold them there for a few seconds and return to the shoulder height

- Repeat 15-20 times

Plank Leg Lifts

If you want an exercise which targets several major muscles all at one time, the plank leg lifts are a great choice. This is a great full-body exercise, but I decided to include it in this section as it is an excellent exercise for strengthening and toning your arms. While performing this exercise, focus on looking forward, rather than down, as it will help you straighten your body and keep your spine as flat as possible.

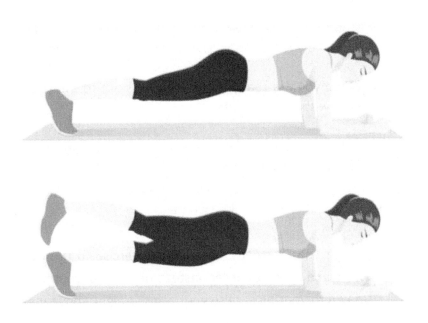

Benefits:

- Ideal for increasing your core strength

- Tones your whole body, especially your legs and arms

- Works out the abdominal muscles

- Stretches the hamstrings and glutes

- Improves your posture

- Burns fat

- Boosts your metabolism

How to do it:

- Lay down on your stomach, bend your hands under your shoulders and lift your body

- Rest your weight on your forearms and the tips of your toes and engage your glutes and the core muscles when doing this

- Lift your right leg to a 45-degree angle and hold for 10 seconds

- Repeat ten times with each leg

Push-Ups

Everyone knows how to do a push-up, but are you sure you are doing them correctly? Push-ups help to boost your upper body strength and again, you simply need a little spare space on the floor to do them.

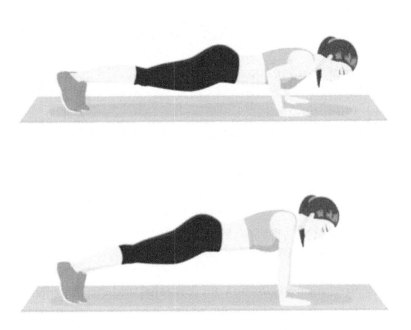

Benefits:

- Works out several major muscle groups, including the triceps, deltoids and pectorals

- Targets your core muscles and helps to build muscle mass over time

- Improves cardiovascular health

- Ideal for overall health and well-being

How to do it:

- Lay down on your stomach and place your hands under your shoulders

- Push upwards into a plank and then extend your arms, so your upper body is higher than your lower body

- Bend your elbows and lower your chest towards the floor

- Push up through your hands to move upwards, straightening out your arms

- Repeat three sets of 10 push-ups

- To make this exercise a little easier, keep your knees on the floor and lower your chest to the mat instead

Chair Push-Ups

If you find regular push-ups difficult, these chair push-ups may help you to tone the major arm muscles and your chest, while making the whole experience so much easier. You will need a chair or a stool to be placed against the wall, or in a position which means it is not going to slip when you put pressure on it. Also, wear shoes as they will give you a better grip.

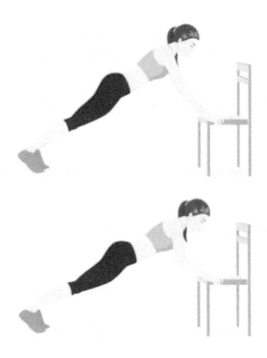

Benefits:

- Targets shoulders and tones the arm muscles

- Great workout for your chest

- A good cardiovascular workout

- Increases strength and endurance

- Helps to improve your balance

How to do it:

- Place your stool or chair in a place where it is not going to slip and put your hands flat on it; keep your legs extended behind you and your body in a straight line

- Raise yourself on to your tiptoes and steady yourself, engaging your core muscles

- Ensure your palms are directly underneath your shoulders, then bend your elbows a little and lower your chest down towards the chair or stool

- Push up through your palms to raise and straighten your arms

- Repeat three sets of 10 push-ups

Triceps Dips with a Bench/Chair

A great bodyweight exercise that helps with building the strength of your arms and shoulders. You can do this workout anywhere; in the park, the kitchen or even in the office. All you need is a bench, a chair or steps.

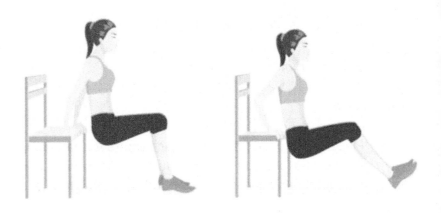

Benefits:

- Works with your chest

- Strengthen the muscles in your triceps, chest and shoulders

- Tones your upper body

How to do it:

- Sit on the edge of the chair/bench and extend your legs hip-width apart, with heels touching the ground

- Look straight ahead with your chin up

- Slide slightly forward and lower yourself down as much as you can or until your elbows are 45-90 degrees

- Slowly push yourself to the starting position and repeat

- Do three sets of 10-15 push-ups and increase it to three sets of 20-30 times over four weeks

- If you find this exercise too hard, then bend your knees and move your feet closer to your body, until you increase your strength and you are able to do it with your legs extended

Lower Body Exercises

Building the strength of your lower body can hugely improve your balance, boost metabolism and reduce pain in your lower back. There are a number of exercises that you can do for your lower back. In this book, I have included the five most common exercises that support your lower body.

Squats

Squats help to tone and strengthen your lower body. If you want to tone your buttocks and thighs, then a series of squats is the ideal option for you.

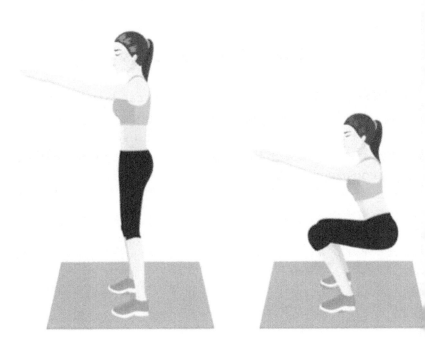

Benefits:

- Tones the buttocks and thighs

- Works out the entire lower body

- Targets the core muscles

- A great cardiovascular workout

- Helps to improve balance

How to do it:

- Stand up straight with your feet in line with your hips

- Keep arms by your side

- Keep your back straight and your chest upwards

- Slowly bend your knees and push your hips backwards

- Your thighs should now be parallel to the floor

- Hold for a second and then push up through your heels to return to your original position

- Do three sets of 12 squats

Lunges

Lunges are a well-known exercise that is ideal for boosting the strength of major leg muscles, but they are also an excellent workout for the heart and cardiovascular system too. The good news is that you only need a little room in your living room to do them!

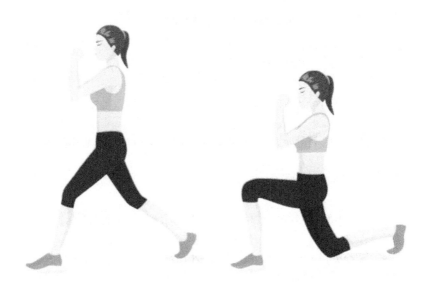

Benefits:

- Works out the major leg muscles, including the hamstrings and quads

- Helps to strengthen and tone the gluteal muscles

- Gives a great cardiovascular workout

- Improves balance

How to do it:

- Stand up straight with your arms relaxed by your sides or have them in front of you like shown in the picture

- Stride forwards with your right foot

- Bend both knees at a 90-degree angle

- Push your power back through your right foot to return to your original standing position

- Repeat ten times on your right leg and another ten times on your left leg

Side Lunges

Side lunges are a great way to work out your abductor muscles. The same as a regular lunge but working to the side instead, just make sure that you have plenty of space around you when you attempt this exercise.

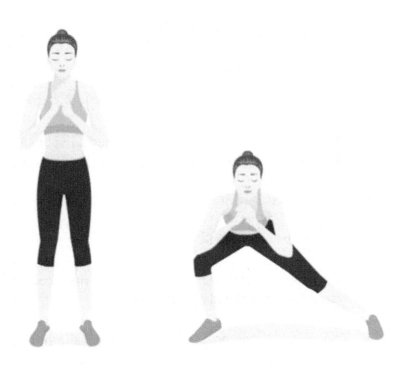

Benefits:

- Works the abductor muscles

- A great cardiovascular workout

- Will help to increase your balance and flexibility

- Works out your core muscles at the same time

How to do it:

- Stand up straight and take a big step to your right side

- Slowly drop down into a lunge so that your right leg is bent at a 90-degree angle

- Keep your left leg straight

- Push through your heel to return to your original position

- Repeat on your right leg ten times

- Repeat the exercise ten times with your left leg

Pistol Squats

If you want to turn up the heat and give yourself the best toning exercise, pistol squats are the way to go. It is a tough exercise, so you may need to take it slowly at first.

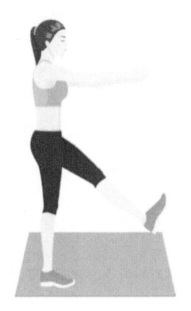 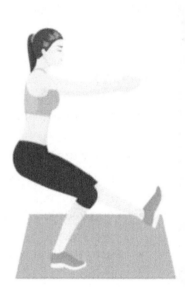

Benefits:

- A great cardiovascular exercise

- Focuses on the quads, hamstrings and the gluteal muscles

- Will add strength to your lower body quickly

- Increases your flexibility and balance

How to do it:

- Stand up straight, with your arms at your sides or in front of you like shown in the picture

- Place your weight on one leg and drop down into a squat, as low as you can go without losing your balance

- As you do, point the other leg out straight in front of you

- Repeat ten times on the same leg

- Switch to the other leg and repeat ten times

Side-Lying Leg Lift

The side-lying leg lift focuses on the lower body and works with many groups of muscles. If you find it too challenging to perform this exercise, you can do the leg lift standing up, instead of lying down. Once you improve your strength, then you can do the leg lift lying down.

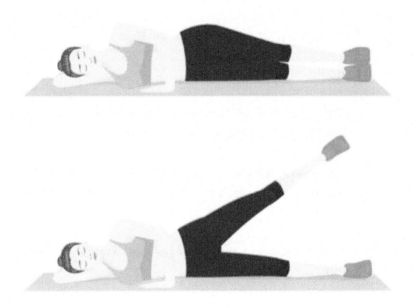

Benefits:

- Focuses on many muscles of your lower body

- Works on glutes, hips, hamstrings, calves, obliques and tights

- Tones your legs, core and butt

- Works with the hip muscles

How to do it:

- Lie down on your side and place one arm under your head and rest the other arm on your hip

- Your top leg should be lying on top of your other leg

- Raise your top leg as high as you can

- Keep your spine straight while doing this exercise

- Lower your top leg down and repeat

- When finished, lie on the other side of the body and repeat this exercise with your other leg

- Start with three sets of 10-15 leg lifts for each leg, until you feel comfortable doing between 20-25 or more lifts with each leg

Strength Training Exercises

Strength training can help your health in many ways. It can make your body stronger, leaner and fitter. It is excellent for your bone health and for improving muscle mass. It offers excellent support to manage chronic diseases such as diabetes, arthritis and cardiovascular disease. It is not uncommon to notice an improvement in energy levels and mood after engaging in a strength training exercise, due to the increased level of endorphins which are released by doing the workout. For weight loss, it is recommended to do regular strength training. Numbers of studies show that strength training can speed up your metabolism, which is responsible for helping manage your weight.

Side Plank

The side plank helps to strengthen your core and abdominal muscles, therefore helping you with your balance and general health and well-being. The side plank is the ideal exercise to try. You might not be able to hold it for too long at first, but the more you practice, the longer you will be able to do it. The side plank will not only add strength to your muscles, but you will also increase your balance and flexibility at the same time.

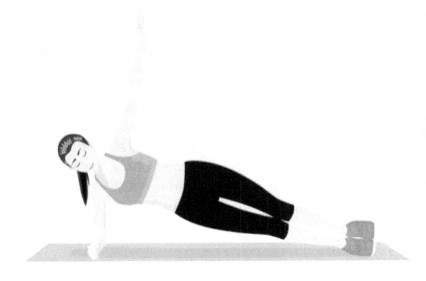

Benefits:

- Works out your core muscles and strengthens all abdominal muscles, including obliques

- Works out your back muscles at the same time

- Great for toning the arms and the inner thighs

- Increases your balance

- Excellent for building your strength in general

How to do it:

- Lay down on one side, put your elbow underneath your shoulder, and place your left foot on top of your right foot

- Keep your feet together and push up your arms and your hips off the floor until you are balancing on your arm and tiptoes

- Hold for a while and relax, before repeating

- If you want to add an extra challenge, try it with a straight arm and raise your opposite arm towards the ceiling, as shown in the picture

- Slowly build up the length of time you can hold the plank

V Sit

You might also hear this called the "boat pose." If you want to give your core muscles the best workout possible, the V sit is a great option. You can initially start holding the V sit for around ten seconds. Then slowly work up to longer increments.

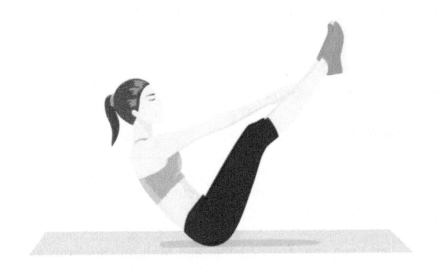

Benefits:

- Works out your core muscles very well

- Focuses on the lower abdominals and the lower back

- Great for working out the hip flexors

- Improves your balance and core strengthen overall

- An excellent cardiovascular workout at the same time

How to do it:

- Lay down on either the ground or a mat

- At the same time, slowly lift your legs (keeping them together) and your upper body, so you form a V shape

- Lift your arms pointing towards your raised legs, to give extra support

- If you want to make it a little easier, bend your legs but raise your feet off the floor

- Hold for ten seconds initially

- Build up to 20 and 30-second increments

Wall Dips

You need to be near a wall for this exercise. You can build up the amount of time you hold the pose for, depending upon how strong you are to begin with. This exercise also gives you a little cardio workout too.

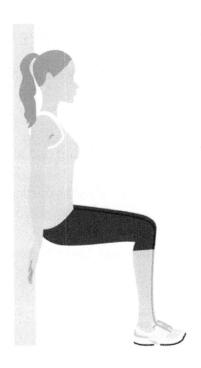

Benefits:

- Works the core muscles and adds strength

- Helps with flexibility and balance

- Gives a cardio element to your workout

- Targets the lower body, including the gluteals, calves, hamstrings and the inner thighs

How to do it:

- Stand up straight with your back against the wall

- Slowly slide your upper back down the wall and bend your legs, so you are in a sitting position

- You should be holding all your weight on your legs

- Hold it for as long as you can, start at ten seconds and build up to longer durations, breath steadily as you go, and repeat a few times

- If you want to make the exercise a little more difficult, get a ball and hold it between your knees

Step up Onto a Chair

This exercise will support you to improve your balance and offer you many health benefits. It is also good for strengthening different muscles in your body. This exercise requires you to have a sturdy chair or a bench.

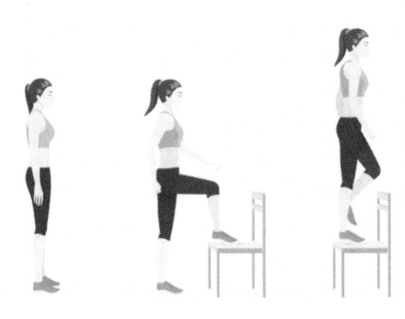

Benefits:

- Exercises the whole body

- Targets the hamstring, quadriceps and glutes

- Tones your legs and buttocks

- Strengthens and tones the entire body

- Helps you to lose weight

- Improves your balance

How to do it:

- Step in front of the chair/bench

- Place the right foot on the chair/bench and then step on it

- Put both of your feet on the floor one by one

- Then repeat with your left foot first

- Repeat as many as you can in 30 seconds

Bird-Dog Exercise

This simple core exercise is excellent for your spine and can support your posture and help reduce lower back pain.

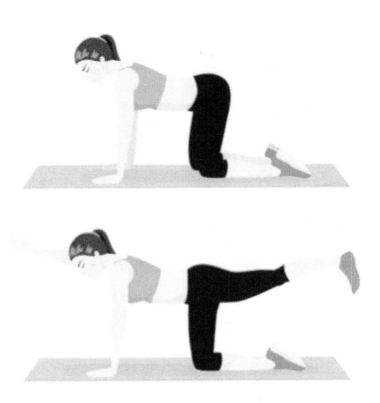

Benefits:

- Strengthens the core and hips

- Works on your back muscles

- Improves your stability

How to do it:

- Get on the floor on your knees

- Keep your spine straight

- Raise your left arm and right leg, keep your shoulders and hips parallel to the floor

- Stay in this position for approximately five seconds and then go back to the starting position

- Then raise your right arm and left leg

- Do two to three sets of 10 times on each side

Stretching

You can do stretching before or after athletic activity or you can do it on its own. There are a number of benefits that you can gain from doing stretching and it is advisable to include it in your daily routine. Stretching is excellent for keeping muscles healthy and strong. Other benefits include improved flexibility, better posture and higher performance in physical activities. It can also help with back pain and relieve stress levels. Stretching helps your body as well as your mind.

Hamstring Stretches

The hamstring muscles are one of the most commonly injured muscles in the body, so it is not only essential to warm them up before exercising, but also to give them a good stretch afterwards. This particular exercise is ideal for that.

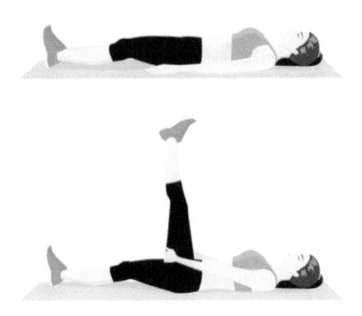

Benefits:

- Works out and stretches the hamstrings

- Increases balance

- A relaxing exercise to finish off your workout

How to do it:

- Lay down on your back with your arms by your sides and both legs fully stretched out

- Start with the right leg first; hold the back of your right knee with both hands and pull it toward your chest

- Slowly straighten the knee until the hamstring feels stretched out

- Keep your back straight throughout

- Hold the stretch for 10-30 seconds

- Repeat with your left leg

Seated Toe Stretches

This is a great stretching exercise that helps with better flexibility. Having better flexibility can improve your mobility and posture. Flexible muscles can decrease the risks of some injuries.

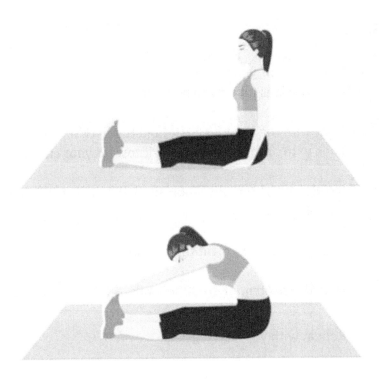

Benefits:

- Improves your physical performance

- Helps with flexibility

- Supports your mobility

How to do it:

- Sit on the floor with your legs straight

- Lift your toes and try to touch them with your hands as shown in the picture

- When you reach your toes, hold for five seconds, and relax

- Repeat 10-15 times

Quad Stretches

If you want to stretch out your quads and increase your balance at the same time, squad stretches are perfect. This can be done before exercise or afterwards, as part of your warm-down.

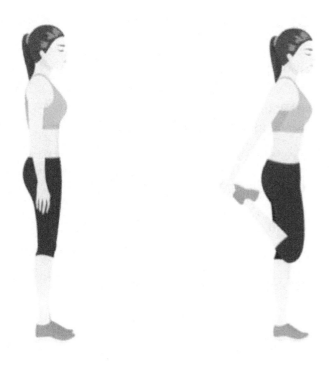

Benefits:

- Stretches out the quads

- Increases your balance

- Improves flexibility

How to do it:

- Stand up straight, with loose shoulders

- Bring your right leg up, bending backwards until it touches your bottom

- Keep your straight leg slightly bent at the knee

- Take hold of your leg with your right arm

- When you are ready and if you want to, push your hips slightly forwards

- Hold the stretch for 30 seconds, then repeat with your left leg

- If you need a little help with balancing, you can hold onto the wall or a chair with your opposite arm

Hip Flexor Stretching

Hip flexor stretching is ideal for you if you are spending long hours sitting down. An inactive lifestyle can cause your hip flexors to become tight and this can cause problems for your lower back.

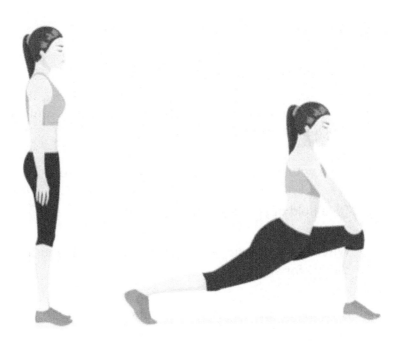

Benefits:

- Can prevent back pain

- Can prevent hip pain

How to do it:

- Get down on your knee

- Place your feet as shown in the picture; one foot is underneath your body, while the other foot is behind you

- Lean forwards while you are squeezing your buttocks

- Hold it for approximately one minute

- Repeat with your other leg

- If you spend long hours every day sitting down, you can do this exercise 2-3 times a day, this will help to prevent pain developing in your hips and the lower back

Bent-Arm Shoulder Stretch

An inactive lifestyle, stress and some physical activities, can cause stress to your body. Most of us tend to hold the most tension in our shoulders, and tight shoulders can cause us to experience pain in our neck, back and upper body. This shoulder stretching exercise can prevent stiffness and help you become more flexible.

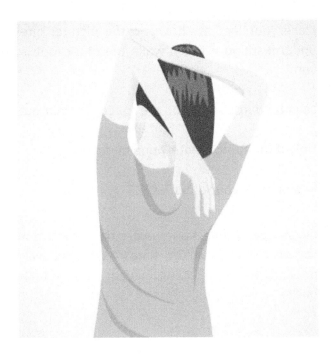

Benefits:

- Stretches several muscles on the side of your upper body

- Stretches your triceps

- Stretches your shoulders

How to do it:

- Stand up or sit down and keep your body straight

- Raise your left arm, bend it to 90 degrees and place it behind your neck

- Use your right arm to gently push the elbow of your left arm behind your back

- Hold the stretch in this position for a minimum of 30 seconds

- Relax and repeat this process with your other arm

Chapter 3: Diet

"A healthy outside starts from the inside."

Rober Urich

Benefits of Healthy Eating

Exercise is vital for good health and weight loss, but it is unlikely to be much of a bonus if you are eating unhealthily.

To lose weight, many people start exercising by going to the gym, running, or engaging in another type of physical activity. However, not many people understand why they are still not losing weight, even though they exercise regularly. An inability to lose weight could be down to a bad diet, an inactive lifestyle, hormonal imbalance, too much stress, or another factor. If you are struggling to lose weight, I cannot confirm the reason for it, but one thing I can confirm is that you cannot out-train a bad diet. To burn off two slices of pizza, you will need to run for at least half an hour. The problem is that not many people settle for only two slices of pizza. They also may have garlic bread, a glass of wine and maybe a dessert. In addition to other foods and drinks consumed throughout the day, this can lead to consuming too many calories in one day.

Healthy eating and exercising should never be only about weight loss. Health must always be your primary focus. I understand that junk food might taste good and that healthy eating can be confusing, hard and even inconvenient for some people (not to mention boring), but those are just unconscious excuses. Once you start eating healthy food, you will not want to go back to your old diet. I would also like to say that in my opinion, healthy food tastes delicious, you just need to know how to prepare it.

Let's look at the benefits of healthy eating. They tend to range from physical to mental benefits. Here are the main ones.

Weight Loss and Disease Prevention

Losing weight is the most common motivation to go on a healthy diet. It can be vital for your psychological well-being since body image has a powerful effect on how happy we are. However, the benefits do not stop there.

Being overweight or obese can increase your risk of many serious diseases and reaching your optimal weight can significantly reduce this risk. Heart disease and strokes, for example, are associated with unhealthy eating and obesity.

Recent research in Canada has suggested that a healthy weight-loss diet can prevent these diseases in 80% of cases.

Similarly, losing weight through healthy eating can help with the management of type 2 diabetes and there is evidence that both a healthy weight and a healthy diet can reduce the risk of developing some types of cancer.

Benefits to the Body's Health

Many aspects of your body need to function at an optimal level for you to be and feel healthy and both these aspects are often significantly improved by healthy eating.

The food you eat is what the body uses to continue building itself, including your bones and teeth. If you ensure your diet includes the various minerals required for this, you are reducing the risk of developing osteoporosis and osteoarthritis in later life.

Similarly, a healthy gut is vital for both health and well-being. A diet rich in prebiotics and probiotics can strengthen the friendly bacteria in your gut, which not only boosts your metabolism, but also fights harmful bacteria and can even reduce the risk of bowel cancer.

Benefits to Mental Health

As mentioned previously, achieving your target weight can have a powerful psychological effect, leaving you feeling much happier and more positive. However, healthy eating can also have more direct benefits on your mood, since some unhealthy foods can contribute to depression and fatigue.

Eating healthy has also been linked to improving brain function. In the short term, this can improve memory, but in the long run, there are suggestions it could also reduce the risk of cognitive decline and dementia as you get older.

If all this is not enough, a healthy diet can also improve your sleep pattern. So, this benefits both your physical and mental health, as well as helping you enjoy a better lifestyle.

What Is a Healthy Diet?

We have established how crucial it is for both your physical and mental well-being to eat healthily. But what exactly is a healthy diet?

According to the NHS, a healthy diet means "Eating a wide variety of foods in the right proportions and consuming the right amount of food and drink to achieve and maintain a healthy body weight." While fad diets are not healthy, they are a type of diet that focuses on limiting food choices and calorie restriction.

What Varieties of Food Should You Be Eating?

There are five primary food groups and all of them are a part of a healthy diet. Some of the foods come from meat or dairy, and if you are either a vegetarian or vegan, there are alternatives available.

- Protein-rich foods, including meat, fish, eggs, beans and pulses, are essential for the body to grow and repair, as well as providing iron, zinc and B vitamins. In the case of meat, poultry is ideal, though lean cuts of other meats are acceptable. I suggest you avoid processed meat as much as possible.

- It is essential to eat at least five portions of fruit and vegetables a day, which can be fresh, dried, tinned or frozen, to provide a range of vitamins and minerals. Vegetables should make up a substantial part of each meal. There is evidence this can lead to a lower risk of strokes and heart disease.

- Starchy foods, which contain fibre, vitamins and minerals, should make up a third of your diet. More natural forms are healthier, like brown rice, whole-wheat pasta, wholemeal bread and potatoes with their skins on.

- Milk, cheese and yoghurt are good sources of protein and calcium, which strengthens your bones. If your diet is dairy-free, alternatives such as soy-based milk and plant-based cheese can give similar benefits.

- Some fat is essential, but make sure you use it in small quantities. Some oils, such as olive oil, are excellent sources of unsaturated fat, which supply the body with fatty acids to absorb vitamins. Saturated fat is not the best option. It usually comes from animal products such as fatty pieces of beef or pork. I want to mention here that coconut oil also contains saturated fat, but as it is a plant, it can provide you with many health benefits. Trans fat can be found in foods such as cakes and biscuits and is the type of fat that you need to steer away from.

Also, it is vital to drink plenty of fluids during the day, the majority of which should be water. Restrict caffeinated and alcoholic drinks to a minimum. Drinking too much alcohol can weaken your immune system and increase the risk of certain diseases such as a stroke, high blood pressure and a heart attack. There are also many side effects of consuming large amounts of caffeinated drinks, which include insomnia, caffeine addiction and high blood pressure.

Eat Sensibly

It is essential to include all these food groups in your daily diet. Some of the foods, such as starch and fat, have traditionally been regarded as causing weight gain. In fact, this is more to do with specific sources, such as white bread and saturated or trans fats. Swapping these for a healthier option in the same group will help towards maintaining your ideal weight.

In general, the fresher and less prepared your ingredients are, the better for you. Although, as noted, frozen or tinned vegetables are often a good substitute. One advantage of preparing meals from scratch is that you always know what is going in them.

This does not mean you cannot eat fast food or a cake ever again, but these foods should be left for specific occasions and used as special treats. Then the following day you can return to your healthy diet again.

What Is the Difference Between a Healthy Diet and a Weight Loss Diet?

We hear a lot about fad diets, but these are the types of so-called diets you need to avoid at all costs. The problem is that many dieters follow this type of diet regularly in the hope that it will help them lose weight.

Some of these diets are extremely dangerous as they do not provide the body with essential nutrients needed for healthy functioning. They tend to focus too much on weight loss and do not pay much attention to health.

To lose weight fast, many people become obsessed with counting calories and this often leads to starvation. So, the weight-loss diet actually turns into a hunger diet.

Generally, weight-loss diets are very restrictive. In addition to removing a fair amount of food you consume daily, dieters also stop eating all the foods they love the most. After doing this for a few days or weeks, dieting becomes a chore that is not sustainable and is very hard to follow. The combination of starvation and deprivation never brings positive results.

It is important to remember there is no such thing as quick weight loss. If you want to lose weight permanently, you need to do it steadily. That means focusing on around 1-2 lb or 1 kg of steady loss every week. You should do this by eating healthy foods, varying your diet and exercising regularly.

A healthy diet is, as we know, a lifestyle choice. It means focusing on clean, natural and fresh foods, lean meats, avoiding sugary foods and high-fat options and steering clear of processed foods. That does not mean you cannot have the odd treat, of course you can, but it should all be in moderation. When you add exercise into that type of lifestyle, you will lose weight, albeit slowly. The plus point of this is that you are more likely to keep the weight off and you will feel far better in yourself too.

There tends to be a big difference between a healthy diet and a weight-loss diet, but it should not be that way. The intention of both diets should be to provide you with healthy nutrients that nourish your body. The issue is that a weight-loss diet often does not do this.

A healthy diet is focusing on the quality of food you consume, while the weight-loss diet is more focused on restricting and minimising the quantity of foods you eat, sometimes to an unhealthy level. When eating healthy, you end up being healthy as well as slim. Therefore, a healthy diet with exercise is always the best route forwards, there is no question about that, whether your goal is to lose weight or to be healthy.

How to Prepare Healthy Meals in Minutes?

In a world that is becoming increasingly defined by complexity and more activity than you can manage to fit into your 24-hour day, it is becoming increasingly difficult to cook a decent meal. We face mounting deadlines and delivery periods that sometimes loom over our heads like a dark cloud.

Some days, you might not even get to eat at all and on other days you may rely on processed foods or start binging on everything from packaged snacks to beverages. While studies continue to point you to the dangers of depending on processed and packaged foods, you see it, but there is nothing much you can do, you think. You want to live healthier, but the speed and mounting pressure that defines your week and life do not allow you to. You have even made plans and resolutions, but the timeline for making that transition from your junk food lifestyle to a healthier living just keeps moving further away.

How to Make a Start

I understand your dilemma, and I can see your difficulties in this regard. However, making a healthy and nutritious meal is not as time-consuming as you have conditioned yourself to believe. With the right meal ideas and different meal combinations to follow, you will very quickly get yourself on a healthy diet while also achieving your deadlines.

Many people believe that eating healthy is expensive, time-consuming or hard to learn, not realising that their lack of knowledge influences these conclusions. If you are one of these people who hold such beliefs, well, then it is great that you are reading this book because you will soon learn that you can make healthy and nutritious meals in minutes. You will find out from the meal ideas I am sharing with you in this book, that living a healthy life lies within your reach and you only need to be pointed in the right direction. The meal ideas in this book are so simple and easy to make. You do not need to be a chef or a great cook to be able to prepare healthy meals and eat healthy. You just need to follow these meal ideas and combine them with the exercises I shared with you in the previous chapter.

Eating Healthy is Not So Hard

You see, nature has provided us with lots of fruits and vegetables. There are over 1000 edible plants that nourish our bodies. There are also various animal proteins and food supplements that can make us healthy and deliver all the nutrients that our bodies need. So, whether you are vegan, vegetarian or love those chicken wings, you can find a space for your appetite. Living healthily does not require you to break the bank or exceed your budget, as the meal combinations and suggestions I will be giving you are both pocket friendly and readily available; talk about having your cake and eating it.

In the next chapter you will find lots of simple meal ideas. They are highly nutritious and focused to get you powering through your schedule while living a healthy life. From breakfast to lunch to dinner and everything in-between, you can combine your need for speed with a convenient meal plan that puts you on a healthy diet and a low budget.

A recipe book *Get Slim and Healthy in 20 Minutes or Less* is yours. It is your free bonus and a great addition to the book you are holding in your hands right now. Go to bit.ly/silvana-recipebook and download your free copy. You will discover lots of healthy and delicious recipes, designed to support you on your journey towards permanent weight loss and good health.

Chapter 4: Simple and Healthy Meal and Drink Ideas

"Good food is very often, even most often, simple food."

Anthony Bourdain

Eating and drinking in a healthy way does not have to be too hard or too confusing. You simply need a few ideas to get you on the right track.

Here are 9 healthy eating tips to get you started and lead you to your success, so you can reach your health and weight loss goals quickly.

Healthy Eating Tips

Start the day with breakfast.
Eat a variety of fruits and vegetables.
Eat lean protein and healthy fats, and try to include them with each meal, if possible.
Consume organic foods whenever possible.
Consume small portion sizes.
Eat frequent meals.
Drink plenty of water.
Do not eat late at night.
Enjoy what you eat!

Simple and Healthy Breakfast Ideas

I am sure you have heard of a famous quote by Adelle Davis, an American author and nutritionist, known for her work in the early to mid-20th century, "Eat breakfast like a king, lunch like a prince and dinner like a pauper."

Since your younger days to much of your adult life, the cliché "breakfast is the most important meal of the day" has been communicated in many different ways. This message remains as important today, as it is correct. As true as it is, however, the most flouted meal of the day is breakfast, and the reason is simple. The mad dash to get out of the door and the daily hustle and bustle of life has effectively made it impossible for many people to have their breakfast, or to put it mildly, a healthy breakfast.

I suggest you try to make some time in the morning to fill your body with the necessary nutrients. Your body will thank you for it. Filling your body with the right fuel at the beginning of each day will help you to feel healthier and more energised. A healthy breakfast will prevent you from reaching for sugary snacks at around 11 a.m. or carbohydrate rich foods for lunch.

Below are some breakfast ideas that would fit into your ever-shrinking time, ensuring that you do not have to skip the most important meal of the day anymore.

Fruit smoothie – Simply place a selection of your favourite fruits into a blender and add a little Greek yoghurt for a healthy and delicious start to your morning. This will kickstart your five a day challenge early on.

Mashed avocado on wholemeal toast – Avocado is packed with vitamins and minerals and it provides your body with healthy fats.

Granola with fruit and yoghurt – Granola will keep you fuller for longer, so you will avoid those mid-morning munchies. Add some berries and a little bit of yoghurt for a delicious and healthy start to the day. Most yoghurts are packed with sugar, therefore I recommend you read food labels. Greek yoghurt is high in protein, so it could be a great choice to have it with your first meal of the day.

Boiled eggs on wholemeal toast – Eggs are a great source of zinc, calcium, protein and all the major vitamin groups.

Wholemeal toast is a slow-release food, so it keeps you full throughout the morning.

Oatmeal with strawberries – If you are not a strawberry fan, you can add any other type of berry and you will be getting a good dose of vitamins and antioxidants, while the oatmeal will fill you up for longer which will prevent you from reaching for an unhealthy snack a couple of hours later.

Vegetable omelette – Use coconut oil, whisk up two eggs and add in your favourite vegetables, such as peppers, onions, tomatoes, mushrooms, etc. Coconut oil will provide your body with healthy fats, while the protein in the eggs will keep you full. You will also receive some antioxidant and vitamin benefits from the vegetables.

Overnight oats – You can have them with a fruit topping: a handful of fresh or frozen berries, grated apple, peach, plum or apricot, or you can have it with a "good" fat topping: nut butter, pumpkin, sunflower seeds, etc.

Pancakes – You can find recipes for a variety of pancakes in the recipe book. Go to bit.ly/silvana-recipebook and download *Get slim and healthy in 20 minutes or less*. Depending on the type of pancakes you go for and the topping you choose (you will notice there is a nice variety there), you will receive many essential nutrients that will prepare your body for the day ahead.

Nut butter with a slice of rye bread – You will receive plenty of healthy nutrients with nut butter including protein, fibre, healthy fat as well as some vitamins and minerals. Due to the high nutrient content it is fine to consume nut butter, but only in moderate amounts. Make sure you do not overdo it because of the high amount of fat in nut butter. From rye bread, you will get plenty of fibre, iron and B vitamins. This can reduce inflammation and help with heart health and it can also support your weight loss.

Two slices of cold salmon, two scrambled eggs and one medium tomato – Salmon provides your body with Omega-3 fatty acids, protein, potassium and B vitamins. From eggs, you will get additional high-quality protein as well as many vitamins and minerals. Tomatoes are rich in antioxidants. Together, these foods will provide you with essential nutrients for your body to function at its best.

Slice of wholemeal toast with three tablespoons of low-sugar baked beans – Beans are a great source of plant-based protein that comes from seeds. They are high in minerals that provide you with energy and help boost your immune system.

Simple and Healthy Lunch Ideas

Lunch happens to be in the middle of the working day for most people. For this reason, many people do not pay much attention to the quality of the food they eat for lunch. They tend to grab whatever they can find in the local shop or a cafe. Here, I am sharing some ideas on what to eat for lunch and it includes a nice variety of food that you can easily prepare at home and take to work.

Lean chicken slices with lettuce, onion and tomatoes – Lean chicken is an excellent source of protein, which keeps you fuller for longer.

Tuna and jacket potato – Stick to a small potato and make sure you cook it in the oven for the best taste. Added tuna is rich in Omega-3, iron and magnesium.

Vegetable soup – Instead of buying tinned soup, I suggest you make it yourself to get the best vitamin content and add in as many vegetables as you enjoy. The more you include, the more vitamins and minerals you will receive and it is a hearty lunch that will keep you full until dinner.

Cauliflower pizza – Did you know that you can make a pizza base with cauliflower? This will make it far healthier from having a flour pizza base. Stick to a small amount of cheese and top with as many vegetables as you want.

Ratatouille – It is high in potassium, folate, fibre and vitamin C. It is very easy to take to work and warm up in the microwave.

Lemon chicken pasta – Stick to wholemeal pasta and grill your chicken instead of frying it for a healthier twist. This meal traditionally has a creamy pasta sauce, but instead of the cream you can add coconut oil and add plenty of vegetables such as spinach, garlic and leaks. The lemon adds a tangy twist and a dose of vitamin C.

Large egg/tuna/grilled chicken salad – This is such a simple and healthy meal idea and it is so easy to prepare. Feel free to choose between the hard-boiled egg, tin of tuna or grilled chicken. Whatever you decide to have as your base, make sure you add a variety of vegetables. Here are some vegetables that you may want to include in your salad: red onion, spring onion, sweetcorn, cucumber, tomatoes, olives, grated carrot, pepper (red, yellow, orange or green), lettuce, spinach, radish, etc. Avoid using a creamy sauce such as mayonnaise or salad cream and instead, use a little bit of olive oil or vinegar. This meal will provide you with plenty of vitamins and minerals that you will gain from vegetables. In addition to this, you will get protein from the egg, tuna or chicken.

Large fruit salad with mixed seeds – Some days you may not be too hungry and having a fruit salad for lunch might be sufficient. Prepare a bowl with chopped pieces of fruits such as an apple, nectarine, banana, grapes, watermelon, etc. and at the end, do not forget to add seeds such as pumpkin or sunflower seeds. Even though the fruits contain natural sugar, it is still a sugar and seeds can provide you with protein, healthy fats, fibre, alongside vitamins and minerals, which will help keep your blood sugar balance stable.

Plain omelette with a large green salad – This simple meal will provide you with all the necessary nutrients: plenty of vitamins and minerals from the salad and protein from the eggs which will keep you full until snacktime or even dinnertime.

Soup – In my recipe book *Get slim and healthy in 20 minutes or less,* you will find a recipe for *Roasted red pepper and tomato soup*. It is easy and quick to prepare and is an excellent choice for a healthy lunch. You will receive all the healthy nutrients from the garlic, tomatoes, almonds, etc.

Wholemeal wrap with tomato, mozzarella and half an avocado – Avocado is a highly nutritious food. It may reduce your chances of developing heart disease and protect you from chronic illnesses, while mozzarella can support your bone health. A wholemeal wrap is a good source of magnesium, potassium and zinc. These vitamins are necessary for the healthy functioning of your body.

Simple and Healthy Dinner Ideas

If you have a long day at work and you are feeling tired by the time you get home, it is so easy to get a takeaway or grab a ready-made meal, or simply buy a sandwich and a bar of chocolate on the way home from work. This is not the best solution and you know it. Therefore, I am sharing with you some simple and healthy meal ideas. They are very easy and quick to prepare.

Jacket sweet potato with your favourite protein filling and green salad – Sweet potato is more nutritious and less fattening than a white jacket potato. It is high in antioxidants and I suggest you eat the potato skin as well, as it is a great source of fibre. Make sure you choose a small sweet potato and add any filling that is rich in protein. It can include tuna, cottage cheese or boiled egg. As a salad dressing, use a sprinkle of olive oil, vinegar or a spoon of squeezed lemon juice.

Baked salmon fillet with vegetables – Salmon is high in protein and rich in healthy fats. It is also high in vitamins and some minerals. Enjoy the fish with green beans, broccoli and three new potatoes.

Grilled fish with roast vegetables – Feel free to choose any white fish and have it with roasted vegetables such as courgettes, leek, peppers and a small portion of cooked brown rice or lentils.

Grilled lean chicken breast with salad – A piece of protein mixed with a few baby tomatoes, half an avocado, plenty of green salad and olive oil as a dressing.

Roasted vegetables – This is a delicious, healthy and easy meal to prepare. You can use the following vegetables: mushrooms, sliced red onions, tomatoes, courgettes, carrots, peppers, herbs, etc. Chop all the vegetables and drizzle with a little oil. When the vegetables are soft, serve them with couscous, which is a great and healthy alternative to pasta or rice. You will receive a high dose of vitamins and minerals to support your overall health. Tip: there is no need to peel courgettes or carrots. Skin of most vegetables is good for you. It will also save you time.

Vegetarian bolognese – Make your bolognese sauce with a small portion of mincemeat and plenty of vegetables. Serve with shaved courgettes instead of pasta. This meal is rich in a variety of nutrients and can help your heart health, digestion and support your weight loss.

Stuffed peppers and brown rice – The brighter the pepper, the higher the antioxidant level and when it is stuffed with brown rice and other vegetables, it is truly delicious. This meal is packed with a variety of vitamins and minerals and the brown rice will keep you fuller.

Garlic stuffed chicken – We all know that chicken is an easy meal and it is a great source of protein, but it can be boring on its own. So, you can cut it in half and stuff it with garlic and cook it in the oven. Garlic is high in iron, calcium, copper and potassium.

Grilled salmon, large salad and new potatoes – Salmon is high in Omega-3 fatty acids, magnesium, zinc and potassium, while also being very filling and delicious. Serve it with large salad and three new potatoes.

Balsamic chicken and asparagus – Simply marinade your chicken in delicious balsamic vinegar for a real kick and add in some asparagus. Not only do you get protein, but you are also getting all the major vitamin groups and fibre from the asparagus.

Eggplant lasagne – Just because you are trying to be healthy, it does not mean you have to give up your favourite food. Eggplant is a great meat substitute, in this case. Make your own tomato sauce and use cheese sparingly for a delicious meal with calcium and vitamins C, K and B.

Simple and Healthy Snack Ideas

Dieters often try to avoid eating a snack but there is nothing wrong with snacking. They will keep you full and satisfied between main meals. The secret is to find what snacks are good for you. Here are some suggestions that will not only satisfy your hunger but will also provide you with healthy nutrients that your body needs. Once again, these are quick, simple and healthy.

Fresh fruit salad with yoghurt – As I already mentioned, you will find that yoghurts tend to be high in sugar. Learning how to read food labels is a must if you want to consume healthy foods. Choose soya yoghurt or Greek yoghurt, which are much healthier options. You can also sprinkle some seeds on top.

Mixed nuts – A handful of nuts can give you a high dose of healthy fats, protein and fibre. Nuts are also linked to a lower risk of heart disease and even prevent certain types of cancer.

Apple slices and peanut butter – Slice an apple and dip it (sparingly) into a little peanut butter. Peanut butter is linked to lowering blood cholesterol and apples are high in fibre. I already mentioned that a small amount of healthy fat is good for you, and you should avoid consuming too much fat.

Kale chips – Kale is super healthy and packed with antioxidants and fibre. You simply need to bake it until crispy.

Cherry tomatoes and mozzarella – From tomatoes, you are getting potassium, and vitamin C, as well as lycopene.

Mozzarella (in moderation) is high in protein and calcium. They are also delicious when combined together.

Hard-boiled eggs – We all know that eggs are very healthy, but they are also a great snack too. Rich in protein, vitamin B12 and K2, eggs will also keep you fuller until you reach lunch or dinnertime.

Olives – Olives can be enjoyed as part of a meal, but they are a great snack too. Olives are also high in healthy fats and antioxidants.

Two Oatcakes with hummus – Rich in protein, fibre and some minerals. They are a great choice to support your weight loss.

Six cubes of feta cheese and six olives – A great source of protein and healthy fats. It will decrease your hunger level between meals and keep your blood sugar levels stable.

Berries with a few nuts – Choose any type of berries and nuts. Berries are high in antioxidants, help with inflammation and are rich in fibre. Nuts are also a great source of fat, protein and fibre, and may also reduce the risk of having a heart attack or stroke.

Spicy nut mix – A great combination of nuts and spices that can provide you with plenty of health benefits. You can find this recipe in *Get slim and healthy in 20 minutes or less*. To download this 29-page recipe book, go to bit.ly/silvana-recipebook.

Simple and Healthy Drink Ideas

The majority of people are aware of what healthy food is, but they are less familiar with what a healthy drink is. So, they may eat healthily, but not drink healthily. Beverages such as Coke, Fanta and most energy drinks are packed with sugar and chemicals not recognisable by the human body and yet people still drink them, often in large amounts. Here are some examples of healthy drinks.

Water with a squeeze of fresh lime and lemon – Even diet versions of your favourite fizzy beverage are high in sweeteners and it is important to keep your body hydrated with as much water as you can. Add a squeeze of fresh lemon and lime to take away the blandness.

Lemon and ginger tea – A little fresh ginger and lemon mixed with hot water will give you a warm and healthy drink. You will get plenty of vitamin C, plus zinc, potassium, magnesium and iron.

Almond milk – Almond milk is a healthier and delicious alternative to regular milk, look for organic options to find the cleanest source possible.

Coconut milk – Coconut milk is a great source of calcium. It also contains magnesium, iron, vitamins C, E and B vitamins.

Turmeric tea – Turmeric is a superfood and contains more than 300 natural vitamins, minerals and other components which are vital for health. It is also delicious and gives you a herby and spicy tea to enjoy.

Fresh mint tea – Fresh mint leaves added to hot water provide a sweet flavour and give you plenty of health benefits, such as improving the symptoms of cold, helping with indigestion and they may also help with inflammation.

Green tea – Green tea is a great detoxing drink, but it is also packed with zinc, manganese and vitamins A to D.

Coconut water – Enjoy the tropical taste and receive vitamin C, B6, folate and plenty of potassium and magnesium.

Smoothie – Choose three different types of fruits, add some seeds and natural water. Mix everything in the blender and enjoy the nutrients that you can find in fruits and seeds.

Chapter 5: Live Healthy Every Day

"Try to think of working out and healthy eating as a lifestyle. Rather than go on a diet or try a crazy exercise routine, try making them something you do every day."

Allyson Felix

How to Establish a Healthy Daily Routine?

Routines are essential for us to function as human beings, allowing us to remember the numerous processes we have to go through in our lives. Routines are made of habits that we repeated over a long period of time and they have a strong impact on our lives. We tend to follow these sequences of repeated patterns without much thought. We do them most of the time on autopilot.

However, due to this it is very easy to fall into routines that could have a harmful effect on our health and lives. Perhaps you have a habit of always buying a chocolate bar or bag of crisps on your way into work. Or maybe you habitually collapse in front of the TV when you get home.

This is the reason why establishing a healthy daily routine is vital to achieving a healthy lifestyle. You need to do it purposefully and for a more extended period, for it to be adopted as part of your life. It is important to understand that working towards establishing your healthy daily routine could be challenging, but it might be necessary to make some sacrifices that will help you to get there.

Establish What You Need to Achieve and What You Need to Avoid

You cannot establish a daily routine unless you know what you want to achieve each day. On the other hand, you also need to know the bad habits you should avoid.

The first step of establishing your healthy routine, therefore, is to make two lists:

1. The things you want to achieve each day
2. The things you currently do that you want to avoid and what you could replace them with

Take a while to think about this and come back to your lists if necessary, in case you do not remember everything the first time.

Your first list must include essentials such as your job, as well as the activities needed for your health — your mealtimes, exercise periods and a good night's sleep. Do not forget to include details about your family time and leisure activities. It is essential to think of things that will enhance your well-being, rather than adding something only because it is easy to do.

Create a Daily Structure

While it is not necessary to assign an exact time for everything, it is useful to group your activities by periods of the day. It might be a good idea to have mealtimes at regular times so you can use them as landmarks. This will help you plan your activities before breakfast, before lunch, between lunch and dinner or after dinner.

Where you place activities like exercise and leisure depends entirely on yourself. Different people are at their best at different times of day, so you may for instance, wish to do your exercise before breakfast or in the early evening.

Routines such as physical structures are likely to break if they are too rigid. It is essential to build in some slack for the unexpected.

For instance, if a crisis prevents you from exercising before breakfast, make sure there is an alternative substitute time for it. Make sure you build-in not only enough time to eat your healthy meals, but also to avoid walking past that vending machine.

Make it part of your routine to take a healthy snack with you, so you are less tempted.

Following Your Routine

At first, it is not going to be easy to remember your new routine, so you will need to be continuously reminded of it. You might find it helpful to have reminders on your phone or put fluorescent coloured stickers on a wall-chart.

Choose something that works well for you.

You might not get it perfectly right every day, especially at first and you should not beat yourself up about the occasional failure. However, it is worth being reasonably strict with yourself, at least initially, so that your healthy routine becomes second nature.

Following your healthy routine is the key to everything I have spoken about in this book.

It is not enough just to have an understanding of healthy eating or planning exercise sessions if distractions or bad habits leave you with no time for them.

Building exercise and healthy eating into your routine is the key. When you are feeling great, physically and mentally, you will wonder how you ever coped without them.

I would like to finish this book by sharing with you the quote from Jim Rohn — American author and motivational speaker.

He is the man behind the famous words, "Take care of your body. It is the only place you have to live."

Life is a journey. Be happy and stay healthy. And take care of your body!

Lots of love XX

Silvana

Conclusion

Having read this book, you now have a straightforward guide on how to get fit and healthy in your own home in 20 minutes or less. As you have seen, there is no great secret about it, just applying some simple principles.

We have seen the crucial importance to your health of both a balanced diet and consistent exercise. Fad diets and pushing your exercise to the limits can actually be damaging, and even at best, they only represent unnecessary punishment for what can be achieved far more simply and enjoyably.

Many of us are motivated to diet and exercise by the desire to lose weight. This is important to your health, but measures you take to lose weight may not necessarily be healthy, whereas if you concentrate on achieving a fit, healthy, and well-balanced body, your weight will normally take care of itself.

We have seen that you do not need a fully equipped gym to get fit or an endless supply of diet food to eat healthily. I have shown you here how you can get fit and prepare healthy meals within 20 minutes in the comfort of your own home.

I have set out a simple 20-minute exercise regime you can follow without requiring any special equipment. This describes routines that allow you to warm up, exercise your upper and lower body and get the benefits of stretching.

In the same way, I have suggested easy but healthy meal ideas and a recipe book for breakfast, lunch and dinner, as well as the snacks and drinks you will need throughout the day. Instead of being based on expensive "diet foods," these meal ideas and recipes use ordinary ingredients that supply the various food groups you need, rather than the unhealthy foods we have been conditioned to reach for.

However, of course, there is no point in reading this book if you do not put its advice into practice. So what can you do now?

Firstly, you can set aside 20 minutes a day and get used to doing the exercise routine I have suggested. If you can, choose the same time each day to do your workout, so it can become a part of your daily routine. At first, you may need to force yourself, but it should quickly become a habit. Once it becomes a habit, you will love your new lifestyle.

Second, planning your meals in advance will help you to stay on track and support your healthy diet. Make sure you factor in preparation time for each meal in your busy schedule. It will take up to 20 minutes to prepare each meal I suggested in this book. Why not download my recipe book to give yourself plenty of ideas? If you have not done it yet, go to bit.ly/silvana-recipebook.

Of course, it is impossible to get everything into a book. If you want to know more about getting fit and healthy, you are very welcome to get in touch with me. I am inviting you to book your complimentary call with me at www.silvanahealthandnutrition.com/booking/.

Thank You

Please consider leaving a review on Amazon – even if it is only a few sentences, it would be a huge help. Here is the link for your convenience. Go to http://viewbook.at/get-fit. Your review will help other readers benefit from the information in this book.

To join the mailing list for updates on future books and to receive information about health, weight loss, and nutrition, please go to bit.ly/silvana-signup.

About the Author

Silvana Siskov has spent many years working with her clients, helping them on the journey towards better health, weight loss and a more enjoyable life. Her passion is to encourage her clients to take action and make changes in their lives, so they can experience more happiness and a better quality of life.

Silvana understands that for many people, weight gain is just a symptom of their bad diet and unhealthy lifestyle. Through her books, she is sharing with readers her knowledge about nutrition and the experiences she has about human behaviour and our daily habits, which influence the direction of our lives.

In her first book *Get your sparkle back: 10 Steps to Weight Loss and Overcoming Emotional Eating*, Silvana looks at the struggles of emotional eaters and the difficulties they face while trying to lose weight. She provides her readers with weight-loss advice and motivates them to overcome their unhealthy eating habits.

In her second book *Live Healthy on a Tight Schedule: 5 Easy Ways for Busy People to Develop Sustainable Habits Around Food, Exercise and Self-Care*, Silvana offers advice and plenty of useful tips to her readers. The guidance that Silvana gives in this book can support readers to live a healthy life, despite being very busy and having demanding jobs and a busy family life.

In Silvana's latest book *Get Fit and Healthy in Your Own Home in 20 Minutes or Less,* she is continuing to help her readers to work towards their health and weight loss goals. Following the advice given in this book, readers can benefit greatly from the meal ideas and home exercises shared in this book.

Silvana's goal is to help as many people as possible to change their unhealthy eating and lifestyle habits, so they can enjoy the benefits of good health and become fitter, slimmer and happier.

Helpful Resources

My Books:

Get Your Sparkle Back: 10 Steps to Weight Loss and Overcoming Emotional Eating

Live Healthy on a Tight Schedule: 5 Easy Ways for Busy People to Develop Sustainable Habits Around Food, Exercise and Self-Care

Get Fit and Healthy on a Tight Schedule 2 Books in 1

Beat Your Menopause Weight Gain: Balance Hormones, Stop Middle-Age Spread, Boost Your Health and Vitality

Free Yourself From Hot Flushes and Night Sweats: The Essential Guide to a Happy And Healthy Menopause

Manage Your Menopause 2 Books in 1: How to Balance Hormones and Prevent Middle-Age Spread

Break the Binge Eating Cycle: Stop Self-Sabotage and Improve Your Relationship With Food

Relaxation and Stress Management Made Simple: 7 Proven Strategies to Calm Your Mind, Stop Negative Thinking and Improve Your Life.

All Books by Silvana Siskov Can be Found at:
http://viewauthor.at/silvanasiskov

Free Mini-Courses:

- Discover 10 Secrets of Successful Weight Loss
- This Is How to Start Eating Less Sugar
- Learn How to Boost Your Energy – 11 Easy Ways
- Your Guide to a Happy and Healthy Menopause
- This Is How to Lose Weight in Your 40s and Beyond

Free Mini-Courses Available at:
www.silvanahealthandnutrition.com/course/

Book Your Complimentary Call With Me at:
www.silvanahealthandnutrition.com/booking/

Made in the USA
Monee, IL
28 March 2022

93691594R00075